Weight!

How did you lose 80 pounds?

William D. Koch

Published by William D. Koch

Copyright © 2014 by William D. Koch

First Edition – January 2014

Chapter 1 The illusion

The most common question I get asked is: How did you do it? I don't give any quick and easy answers, but I do provide my casual inquisitors with a summary. I briefly describe my eating patterns and my exercise programs. But my answers – in a sense – don't seem to satisfy them. Simply put and for brevity's sake, I say I eat less and exercise more.

But that's the oversimplified version of my weight-loss program. I tell them I have names for the program, and people often say they've never heard of that program before. And I tell them that I just made it up. And that's why they've never heard of it. I call it the "bite" diet. Or I call it the "Bill" diet. And unless you have some time on your hands, I say, that's it in a nutshell.

I get these questions frequently. How did you do it? I finally decided I'd write it down that way I won't have to explain it. The inquiries are constant – at least for people who saw me nine months ago. I weighed 280 pounds.

I had convinced myself – despite having pants with 44-inch waist sizes – that I was just big boned. Yea, that's it. And besides, looking at my shape straight on in the mirror I could conceivable convince myself that I wasn't really "fat." I'm just husky.

I used to go to the gym. I'd ride the stationary bicycle; I'd walk on the treadmill. I'd lift heavy weights. And hey I even ate relatively healthy. (Not really.) I was invincible. I was strong. I was in shape. It's just that the scale unfairly displayed 280 whenever I stepped on it – a gross injustice in the larger scheme of this weight-loss universe. I merely had the inconvenient and inglorious struggle of having to ignore the misguided and patently offensive ruling of the scale – and of course the round belly that hung over my belt.

But looking back from a distance, I recognize the deception. I wasn't husky. I wasn't merely big boned. I was fat. Fat, fat, fat. I see overweight people who weigh more than 250 pounds. They are not big boned. They are not merely a few pounds over weight. They are fat. Like I was.

People ask me if there were any particular events that motivated me to begin this program. I really can't pinpoint any. For the sake of empty conversation and to accommodate the person who asked the question, I mention a visit to a gym in another city. Accustomed to going to gyms, I entered this one and was told that, besides paying the visitor entry fee, I had to have my blood pressure tested. Not a problem. Sorry, I was told. You can't work out. You're blood pressure is too high.

Too high, I protested. I work out all the time. I'm in better shape than most of these people here. Well, except for being 280 pounds. I was never able to work out at that gym. I returned later one more time. And my blood pressure was still too high.

The doctor told me I'd have to take blood pressure medication. Or lose weight. Well, sure. I'd lose weight, I told him. But I never did. I did minor dietary changes. I'd eat yogurt instead of ice cream. I'd have more chicken curry instead of the greasy egg rolls. I'd drink diet instead of regular soda. I'd even ride the gym bicycle longer and harder. But 280 pounds and 44 inches appeared here to say.

So, really, there was nothing that marked the change, except perhaps an epiphany of sorts. It happened in January. I came to the realization that I could lose weight. That drastic, healthy weight loss was a real and attainable pursuit. Over the course of several weeks, I developed what in a sense is a program. And I labeled it the "bite" diet because people kept asking me how I was doing it.

Chapter 2 The delusions

I was sitting in the sauna at the gym one day in early February. An average-sized man was describing to a young woman the secrets of weight loss. He provided her with the standard tenets of the religion of modern dieting – most of which have all become cliché and overstated.

Don't become a slave to the scale, he opined. The scale will discourage you, he said. The scale will frustrate you. He told her to weigh herself only once a week. She listened attentively to his advice. I later learned that the man had never lost a significant amount of weight. He may have lost 10 pounds at one time. But he was never really overweight. His knowledge was based on conventional wisdom. Surf the internet and you're sure to come up with sundry solutions for how to lose weight and get in shape. Quick and easy.

Television offers so many programs. Buy this, eat this, do this. And to convince you even further, here are the testimonials. This woman lost 50 pounds. This woman lost 80 pounds. The stories are probably true and the programs probably work. But becoming part of a program involves investment and commitment, both of which are vital to success. The programs do generate results. But how many of us are willing to take that extra step when being overweight is sometimes so easy to ignore? We can ignore the sad fact of our conditions because we rarely have to see it or confront it – until we are shown photographs of ourselves.

Sometimes the realization strikes us: I really am fat. But the impression often doesn't resonate for long. It fades or we drive it away with other of life's excursions, such as eating. But weight loss is not about where we are but where we can be. Weight loss is about realizing we can reach our potential. Our weight-loss goals are attainable. That's the first thought that we allow access into our heads – that we can be slim. We can reach our goals.

Chapter 3 The path

Years ago, I raised my hand in a college biology class and asked a question that I later learned had more to do with chemistry. The professor said, "KISS. Keep it simple, stupid."

The internet, books and television are packed tight with information about losing weight. Do this, they say. Don't eat this. Cut these foods out. Many of us may already be familiar with the plethora of facts and programs about dieting, exercising and developing fine physiques. Experts direct their audiences down so many different behavioral and lifestyle paths that the way to losing weight can become confusing, troubling, too much of a hassle.

Sticking with an effective program involves more than just raw disciple and determined desire. We have to change the way we think about food and what we eat. And while that doesn't come easily, taking the first few steps to a physical transformation is easy.

This book is not about what you can and cannot eat. It won't tell you to count calories or stay away from salt or sugar or coffee. But what it will do is hopefully lead you to more healthy and productive habits. The best motivator for losing weight is, after all, losing weight; it's seeing results. It's getting on the scale and seeing a downward change.

The man in the sauna who said don't became a slave to the scale was wrong. My first advice is, simply, become a slave to the scale. Use it every day. Twice a day maybe. Once in the morning and once in the evening. The readings the scale gives you have to play a prominent role in your everyday life. Write the numbers down on cards or on your cell phone. The numbers have to be in a place where you can see them often. You have to lodge them securely and tightly in your daily memory banks. Write the numbers on cards and include your record low weight and your monthly goal weight.

The cards should include three numbers: Your current weight, your record low weight and your monthly goal weight. I advise putting the numbers on your notepad on your cell phone – in some other very visible place – so that you are able to access and see the information often. You'll be able to tell what your weight is exactly at any time.

Knowing your current weight serves as sort of a trainer or task master – reminding you that if you keep on eating you're putting distance between your goal weight and your present weight.

That serves to encourage you or frustrate you. Either way, you're focusing on your goal. Many of us have the habit of rewarding ourselves with eating. Knowing you've broken through to a new low in weight loss over time creates a new habit. The scale rewards us. The scale applauds us. And sometimes the scale rightly reprimands us.

The scale makes weight loss existential – in the same way that eating does. We eat in the now. And we lose weight in the now.

Effective weight loss is about recognizing when weight loss is happening. I believe it happens when my stomach is empty – or at least it feels empty. That stomach growling shouldn't serve as the constant, spoiled beast demanding and receiving satiation. The feeling of an empty stomach should be embraced – sometimes – as the state in which weight loss is occurring. We gain weight or stay fat when our stomachs are continually fed. An empty stomach means something potentially good is taking place.

Don't let the monster of empty stomach dictate to you when and what you should eat. And don't let feeding an angry stomach serve as a panacea for what's ailing you emotionally. Too often we reward ourselves for jobs well done with food or assuage tough times or difficult circumstances with food.

We have to change that mindset. We have to keep in mind the rewards for reaching goals is that number on the scale. We have to keep looking forward. We have to keep watching the numbers because the numbers will provide the reward. I'll discuss this more in detail in later chapters.

Chapter 4 Open wide

I use the notepad on my cell phone to keep track of my progress. Once again, the key to success is keeping your plan simple. And don't forget. You have to have a plan. You cannot just have a strong desire or be merely determined to lose weight. Without a plan – and goals – you are setting yourself up for failure. That's the reality of losing weight.

The first number that I list is my most recent weight. That's the number the scale displayed this morning. It's the most important number to keep in mind throughout the day. What do I weigh right now?

The second number is my short-term goal weight, which I'll discuss more in depth later. You're usually within ten pounds of reaching that number. The difference between those two numbers is important. Hopefully, it remains a single digit and continues to drop. But if it rises and goes into the double digits, keep it there. Don't delete or erase it. Let it serve as a negative motivator. You're off target. Straighten up your act.

The third number is your record low weight and the date you reached it. In your program your weight may fluctuate. You may gain weight, but the record-low weight offers some encouragement.

Keep this information with you at all times (in your wallet or purse) and in some other visible locations – even for others to see. The numbers should haunt or inspire you. They should depress or impress you. The numbers have to be with you constantly as your psychological companion. The man in the sauna didn't lose weight. He just had advice that he had heard about losing weight.

The numbers may read something like this: "Current: 250. Record low: 248 on Jan. 16. January goal: 246."

In this KISS diet, it's not what you eat. It's about how much you eat. There's no calorie counting. There's no buying a special diet. There's no protein loading or eating more fruits and vegetables. (Maybe later if you choose.) Good and healthy eating habits will come, and they will come slowly and naturally. This is the "bites" diet and you have to monitor how much you eat – specifically, how many bites you eat.

I started with 50 bites a day. It forces you to monitor what you eat and it compels you to slow down. And a bite is just a mouthful of food. If you're going to cheat yourself with big bites, you can lessen the number of bites. But honestly eating 50 bites roughly equates to less than 2,000 calories on average per day. That's enough for a man to lose about two pounds a week. A woman should drop it to 40 to 45 bites. But you determine how many bites, and once you reach that number, you're done for the day.

Over time, you'll start figuring you have to limit how much you have at breakfast. That is if you don't want to get hit by intense hunger pangs later in the day. But even if you do, being hungry is a good sign. Set a reasonable number. You shouldn't set bite numbers below 30 bites a day.

During hungry times, acquire another habit. I started chewing gums. I've almost become a connoisseur of gum chewing. I have my favorite gum and favorite flavors.

The unusual part of this diet is you begin to look for more dense and – by happenstance – healthier foods. I've started eating pickles, olives and crackers, a food taste I have never had before. In the past my idea of diet food was yogurt instead of ice cream.

My shopping habits have over time changed. I shop differently. To fulfill my set bite allowance I have to find food at the grocery store that better fills my appetite. I've learned to stay away from certain foods, not because I have to, but they hinder the downward weight progression. And that's a discussion for the next chapter.

Chapter 5 Reach this goal

Goals are important. You have to set numeric goals that serve as benchmarks. As you lose weight, you have to follow a predetermined path – in the same way as daily weighing. I've set monthly goals by marking my cell phone calendar on the last day of the month. If weight loss moves unsteadily or inconsistently, I've set weekly goals which coincide with the monthly goal. I'd suggest a weight-loss plan which will not exceed ten pounds a month. And mark the calendar 12 months ahead – that is, if you have that much to lose.

You could set five-pound drops per month. Determine your current weight and mark the calendar for the end of the next month. That way if you're getting close to the middle or the end of the month the decline isn't so radical. As mentioned earlier, commit your current weight for the day and your end-of-month goal to memory. You go through your day with those two numbers in your head.

Ideally, you have to keep in mind that you don't want to lose that much more than the two or three pounds a week. But two pounds adds up to nearly ten a month and you're well over 100 pounds in a year. Numbering is significant because it is precise and current. The daily number won't change over the course of the day. Keeping your number in mind helps shape over time the way you eat.

As your weight declines, you learn to recognize the patterns. This diet is about shaping your own program in your own mind. So, feel free to modify numbers, change goals, incorporate different approaches. Following a rigid regiment someone else has set conditions you to rely on that individual's program. This enables you to create your own. It's about ownership.

On the other hand, you have to establish a program that requires you to develop discipline.

You will likely fail if you rely merely on the force of your individual will power. In other words, you have to follow a rigid, disciplined program that you have had direct involvement in developing for yourself. It has to be personal and geared toward your needs and schedule.

This self-styled program focuses your attention on your progress and serves as a sort of personal in-built trainer. Weight fluctuations happen which will sometimes force you to make adjustments. That might require you to shift your monthly weight loss goals slightly or it might require you to step up your plan to force yourself through a plateau. But it's your program. You are accountable to no one or to nothing except that scale and its blunt sequence of numbers. And if it's a good scale, it won't lie or cheat. It'll be brutally honest with you and hopefully force you every morning to make the daily adjustments you need.

You'll learn over time that certain foods – in my case, peanuts – serve only to sabotage your downward trajectory. You'll learn to recognize over time that the obnoxious scale, bearing for too long the same old bad news, refuses to budge because of a certain "innocent" food. You learn to identify that food and stay away from it.

I developed a list of foods I try to stay away from: peanuts, sweets, soda and candy. Recently, I've discovered that I can't keep drinking the same beverages – the rich coffees – that I've always had. The "bad" foods gain a certain prominence in your mind and you have to find alternatives. You learn to condition your mind and shift your attention away from certain foods. You have to develop a most unwanted list.

You'll always have certain cravings, but over time the temptations diminish, little by little. Healthier foods become more attractive and enticing. You are not pushing yourself away from unhealthy choices necessarily – against your will because of the requirements and demands of your diet – but you are actively choosing to eat healthier. Therein lays the benefit. Changing your mind about food choices leads you to healthier habits. And it generally happens over time. The habit settles onto you and you begin to connect more with the results – the declining weight – than with the momentary satisfaction of eating.

Your plan also focuses you on your diet. Increasingly your attention is placed on goals – both short-term and long-term – rather than filling your stomach. That's why knowing what you weigh at any particular time – especially when you are gazing into a vending machine or are staring at a menu – helps to keep your plan in mind. You're less apt too indulge if you know how much you weigh presently, how much you used to weigh and how much you hope to weigh tomorrow morning and at the end of the month. Losing weight becomes mental. It becomes, hopefully, a contest between your will and your body. And the more weight you lose the more confidence you'll gain in the process.

The task of losing weight must rise to a new level in your life. It must become something that consumes you. It must become almost a part-time job, something that is with you all the time. It cannot be merely an excursion you set to the side and only bring out during discouraging times. You have to go after your weight goals with enthusiasm. You have to drive to your goal and learn to recognize the signs and the directions to reach your destination. It's not an easy route. And there's no simple way to get there. You have to wrestle with two strong desires and biological systems. One obviously is the desire to eat.

You've undergone so much conditioning in the years it took to gain the extra weight. Now you have to unravel that conditioning and establish the training to make the changes. You have to adopt new habits that will rewire your psychological circuits so that you don't end up right back where you started. The rewards are great, but the pitfalls and the discouragement are real, and you have to learn to recognize them, do battle with them and get past them.

It isn't easy. The fight to turn around your weight won't be without struggle. But to reach your goals you need to eliminate as many barriers as possible. Making it simple and easy – at least concerning your plan's organization – will make the way smoother. The straight path to weight loss will take you to your goal, but the route may ascend sharply at times.

You have set your mind to the task. You wade through your life and remove temptations. Over time the lure of certain foods will lose their power. All temptations won't go away entirely, and the ideal isn't to eat stridently and to maintain an austere diet. Our environments and our circumstances make that scenario difficult. The aim is to release yourself from the dependence on certain foods, such as sweets.

Moderation is the key, but moderation for the sake of moderation won't work. It may be acceptable to indulge at times, but the balance comes in realizing that you'll have to pay the price later on. Slowly you'll learn that eating two bowls of ice cream isn't worth the skimping you'll have to do later.

The key is you are in charge of your diet and you – and the scale – are the one you have to face. It's not, in and of itself, about external programs or plans – high protein, low protein, ten meals a day – it's about finding what works for you. And from there comes the attitude.

Chapter 6 The right attitude

Reaching your goal involves developing an attitude. You cannot simply have a strong will or determination. You have to have an attitude. And that attitude is that nothing will stop you from reaching your weight goal. Nothing's going to get in your way.

Before losing weight, you have to develop the mindset that will push you through the setbacks, the fluctuations, the temptations and the distractions. Along the way, you'll gain confidence as you see the pounds drop, but you'll also experience discouragement. You'll hit weight plateaus that may appear impassable. That's where your attitude – finely tuned and built strong – comes in and helps you to hold on.

During discouraging times, you have to remember – you have to keep reminding yourself – that these are just a lull in the downward descent. You have to be strong and remind yourself consistently and repeatedly of your overall goal. You have to maintain your vision and feed off the encouragement and the confidence you've built up along the way.

Discouraging times in your program will come to shake your resolve, but the secret is to employ your newly created attitude. Getting to your ideal weight – reaching that goal – has to become a part of your everyday vision. It may be a long trek (50 or more pounds) or it may be a short trip (lose 20), but it's your determination in the face of so many obstacles (and temptations) that will get you there.

It's a fight. But the rewards are worth it. And as the fight commences, the struggle gets easier. You get used to the confrontations, the temptations and the urges. You'll begin to recognize the habits and eating patterns that cause the most trouble. You'll also learn to adopt healthy habits and to consume diet-friendly foods. You'll engage the enemy (those enticing and heavily armed with empty calories) and you'll begin to make battlefield alliances (those calorie lean, muscled and nutritious items).

As you progress, you'll be adopting a fighting attitude. You'll be determined and you'll refuse to give in to the enemy's traps along the way. The saboteurs of your diet won't confront you head on, but will engage you from the side, from the rear, during your weak moments. As a health soldier, you'll begin to become aware of those dietary attacks and you'll recognize the assaults,

The battle wages in your mind – as it receives signals from your stomach. Your body sends signals – the empty, growling stomach and the exorbitant cravings – and you'll learn to counter those offensives. As the war wages, the victories are measured in pounds. The long-range conquests are measured in inches; clothing sizes drop and clothing gets looser. It's that long view of the effort you have to hold. It's the struggle you'll have to embrace.

To me it's mostly a waste of time and money to employ external weapons – fancy and sometimes expensive fad diets and special supplements – to fight the weight-loss battle. You have to lay out your plan, set your goal and settle in for the fight. And hang on as you take battlefield after battlefield.

As in war, setbacks inevitably come, but those are just the small battles in the overall war. You are the general. You are the commander in chief.

This is your body, and no one else can lose the weight for you. But more about this, too, will come later.

Losing weight is essentially about reducing calorie intake – about 80 percent – and increasing calorie expenditure. So, while exercise is good, the bulk of your energy has to be spent on the largest part of the plan. The next chapter will deal with exercise, an essential component in your program.

Chapter 7 Get moving

Exercise is important – for obvious reasons. It must become an integral part of your plan. Without it your chances of winning the weight-loss war diminish. But exercise should not be overemphasized. Some shift their focus on exercise as the great panacea. They take exercise – as some have with their diets – to intense and complicated extremes. You may discover, as many dieters have, that spending hours in the gym will not get you to your goal more quickly.

Only about 20 percent of weight loss comes from exercise. That's a sizeable amount, and without a diet plan it's unlikely you'll reach your benchmarks. Exercise must be coupled with diet in a consistent manner.

The key to incorporating exercise in your diet, according to my plan, is in the same way you develop a diet program. You keep it simple, but you keep it consistent, regimented and regular. You exercise by units, and you establish modest, easily reachable exercise goals.

Exercise isn't so much about the exertion as the conditioning of the mind to accept routine movement as a regular part of your schedule. And one of the simplest exercises is walking. And when I say walking I don't mean just a casual stroll, and I don't mean race walking either. Find an exercise, and I think walking is ideal, and do it.

The key elements are to make exercise – or walking in this case – a daily routine and tie it to your schedule. Walking must become as regular a habit as, say, brushing your teeth. You cannot go to bed unless you do it. This is where the minimums enter the plan. With the diet portion of the plan, you set maximum daily bites of food per day. With this exercise portion, you set minimums. And make it simple and easy. Don't be afraid to set it too low and avoid – at least for several months if you're a beginner – the inevitable temptation to increase the minimum. That temptation can put exercise plans on indefinite holds. You get a boost of fitness, raise the minimum daily exertion requirements, then you fall back to previous fitness levels and frustration sets in. That's when you quit.

With exercise, as with diet, you have to learn to recognize the tricks and the devices your body will use to get you to stop. Quitting is easy and is the natural reaction of your physical body. Exercise, while vital to your weight-loss plan, is far more a matter of the mind, and the greatest obstacle for long-range benefits is overcoming the initial sense of over confidence you may gain at a certain level. This applies mostly to newcomers. Your body goes through peaks and valleys, but exercising is a contest mostly of the mind, which indirectly and ultimately benefits the body.

That's how you have to approach weight loss – as a battlefield in the mind. You have to wage war against cravings and habits long bred into your psyche. Over time the mind establishes new patterns and cravings begin to change. Naturally, you learn that feeling satisfied after eating doesn't take large quantities of food.

Conventional wisdom about the stomach sending messages to the brain that it's been adequately fed is true. I think researchers say it takes about 20 minutes for that to happen. But that's not the point or aim of this diet. Forcing yourself to wait an allotted time only adds another layer – another level of dietary bureaucracy – to the mix. And rules and regulations complicate the plan and can slow the progression to your goals.

Weight loss has to move simply and steadily, but that doesn't mean you won't encounter some biological resistance. You have to clear the way of as many mental obstacles as possible to make your way straight – the fewer the hindrances the greater the prospects for smooth weight loss.

Set for yourself minimum daily exercise segments. That may entail something as easy as walking around the block. You can set a minimum of five minutes of walking. And, as I mentioned earlier, don't give in to the temptation to go above that amount for at least six weeks. Over confidence is a trap that can lead to injuries and frustration. Remember, this is about laying a new psychological line in your mind. You're establishing a new habit and that requires time.

Simple exercises – walking, riding a bicycle, going to the gym for a short work out – help to lay new mental circuits. The goal – accomplished subconsciously, so to speak – is to make you enjoy exercise, to incorporate it as a mandatory part of your life. Your everyday thoughts and motivations follow certain neural routes, so equipping your brain with new paths that benefit you moves you closer to your real objective of losing that extra weight.

The worst-case scenario is that, even if you don't lose the weight or you give up, you've acquired a very healthy habit. Again, dieting and exercising are head games, and mere acts of the will hardly bring you to your desired end. You have to get into your head and do some rewiring. You have to change circuits and redirect signals so that your brain does all the work. You become by nature a weight loser by naturally gravitating to habits that are helpful.

This isn't to suggest that you cannot step away from your diet and splurge. An occasional detour isn't a catastrophic event. Succumbing to temptation produces less dramatic consequences over time. Rather than sneaking two bowls of ice cream you indulge on a half bowl. Oops. You've slipped up, but there's no need to scrap the whole program.

But back to exercise. Tie the effort to an already ingrained habit such as, for example, brushing your teeth at night. You cannot brush your teeth before bed until you've done your exercise. No excuses. Pouring rain, blizzards, hurricanes, tornadoes. You have to find a way to do the deed. That's why it has to be simple.

You can't have a way out. Once you make one excuse on one day, you can find an excuse for any other day. Plus, once you go walking in the dark, late at night, in the cold or rain, you'll begin to learn you'll have to change your daily routine to prevent yourself from doing it again. You can't allow any excuses – even if it means walking around your living room 100 times.

Think about your daily habits. It doesn't take much mental effort or exertion to do those things that are part of your daily routine. You look in the mirror. You comb your hair. You shower or bathe. You brush your teeth. They are small physical habits that require little thought or persuasion and you would probably allow few or no excuses to compel you to abandon the habits.

Attaching a new habit shifts the weight of the load to an established mental path. You may give in to the temptation to forego an established habit to avoid the newly acquired habit. So be it. However, every action carries a consequence. Do you really want to give up brushing your teeth or bathing every day?

If you're that stubborn, tie your exercise habit to a weightier routine. You cannot bathe until exercising is completed. You cannot eat until you exercise. If it's not working, keep increasing the ante. Keep raising the stakes. And it's not difficult. You are merely training your mind to get accustomed to the habit of exercise so when you start the routine, it should be easy, even insignificant. You're really convincing your mind that moving your body is an acceptable, convenient and easy task to manage. You are, in effect, attempting to outwit yourself into believing that you habitually exercise.

It won't take long. And you should allow the habit of exercise to become a part of life and routine slowly. Moving your body to burn calories is a mixed bag – and some people find the relationship with exercise invigorating at first. Exercise gives them confidence, and they acquire a new-found sense of vigor.

Their exercise routine becomes a passion, a love affair of sorts. But therein lay the danger. Allowing exercise to become a part of your life is very significant and transformative. But the different feelings a beginner gets in the early stages can be misleading. You have to learn to read the signals your body sends after you reach those new levels of ability. You cannot afford to misread the early signs – the risk of burnout and sudden lost of interest is real.

You have to use exercise to suit your needs and goals. That means you have to keep it steady and take it easy. You should increase exercise levels gradually and resist the temptation to increase the load too early. It's sometimes better to keep exercise levels at annoyingly easy levels once your body starts reconditioning itself.

You will experience a surge in energy, but you have to recognize that desire to exercise more may lead you to injury or apathy. You have to keep in mind, especially in the beginning, that your exercise routine is more about mental movement than physical movement. The idea of exercise should fade into the subconscious recesses of mind until it becomes so natural that you wouldn't think of not exercising. You exercise because you can exercise. You exercise because you wouldn't have it any other way. You wouldn't think twice about foregoing exercise. You exercise because that's what you do. It has to become that simple – mentally.

Another part of exercise is to remember you can break it up into segments. You don't have to do all your daily exercise all at once. But you do have to finish your daily allotment by the end of the day. This means that if you designate, for example, ten minutes of walking every day, you can do five in the morning and five in the evening. Or you can do four in the morning, four at noon and two at night.

After you increase your exercise levels, you may want to break up your routine to fit a busy schedule. But again beware of establishing an overly ambitious schedule. My advice: Take it easy. And keep at it. The best way to accomplish this task is to get a watch with a timer. Set the timer to your daily minimum at the start of your day and the only way to finish the day is for the allotment to go to zero – while you exercise. You can't run the timer if you're idle.

Twenty minutes can be broken into as many smaller segments as you like. Or you can do it all at once and get it out of the way. The watch with the timer works with you in the same way the weight scale does. It motivates or discourages you – as a personal trainer would do, except the watch is with you all the time.

You wear the watch and the scale waits for you in the morning and the evening. Let them work for you. Use them as tools to reach your weight goal. Your calendar with the weight goals also helps to keep you on track.

But there's wiggle room in my system – at least involving timing of the exercise. You have to determine the set amount you will go per day. Once you complete it, you can write in your log or on your to-do list that it's completed for the day. But you have to complete the entire allotted time. You cannot hold over any time. But what you can do is go into tomorrow's time. That technically means – for the extra work – you'll have less time the next day. Here's how it may look: You determine that you'll go, in the beginning, 15 minutes per day. You set your watch timer to 15 minutes. But today, for example, you have a little more energy and you do the 15 minutes and another five minutes. The five minutes is taken from tomorrow's tabulation. Tomorrow you only have to go ten minutes.

But there's a catch. You can only advance by one day. You cannot do 60 minutes hoping that you won't have to do any for the following three days. At the 15-minute level, you can only go 29 minutes; that's the maximum. Anything more is off the books. The crucial part of this plan is that you're exercising every day, no matter what and no matter how little. The 29-minute day allows you to have a 1-minute day. That's the wiggle room. You work hard on one day, and you can reward yourself on the next day. But you still have to walk every day. Remember. Exercise is mental. You have to get it in your head first before it translates to your body.

Another part of your exercise routine, which is optional, is incorporating muscle movements.

This may include pushups, sit ups or weight training. I don't think this should be mandatory, but I would encourage considering making it part of your routine. And if you do decide to include this type of exercise, institute it in the same way as your aerobic portion. It too has to become habit. All physical exercise should be tied to an already established activity of your life.

Find a few key exercises you can do easily and adequately, and incorporate them into your daily life – in a psychological way. For instance, if you decide you're going to start with pushups, decide you're going to do three sets of them per day. And that's it. You don't have to do them all at once, at the same time. You can do one set in the morning and two in the evening. A set is one group of repetitions. You get down and do ten of them. That would be a set. The number of repetitions should be predetermined. Doing ten pushups, for example, shouldn't be a breeze. You should be exerting yourself during the final few repetitions. As you improve, you can increase the number of sets per day – but slowly. Resist the temptation to increase by leaps and bounds.

If you decide to do all of your sets at once, that's acceptable. But, if you do, you may reduce the number of required repetitions per set as you tire. For example, do 10, then eight then six. The important part is to determine a daily minimum. If you enjoy the exercises and feel motivated, you may add to the weekly total, but not to the daily.

Here's why and how. Let's say you set a minimum weekly total of 30 sets of exercises per week. Then you set the daily minimum at a tenth of the weekly total. That means you have to do at least three sets per day. But some days you may want to do more – and that's important to set aside days when you do extra. On a high-energy day, you do 15 sets. That leaves a total of 15 for the rest of the week, which means you can take it easy. But you still have to do the minimum of three per day.

Here's another scenario, using the same numbers. Your weekly total is 30. You do the minimum of three for the first six days for a total of 18. On your last day you have to do 12 to fulfill your week's number. Or, you can do five per day and take it easy on the last three days. The point is this plan is to get you used to do something everyday, but allow some leeway.

The plan is simpler than it may sound. You're dealing with weekly maximums and daily minimums. That's about it. Once you get a hold of the concept, it allows you some room throughout the week but forces you to do some activity every day. The plan propels you.

The next chapter deals with ways to alleviate those inevitable hunger pangs that follow.

Chapter 8 Supplements

I take supplements. I have taken supplements most of my life. I found the science behind the need for nutritional supplementation fascinating. Some experts purport that we need to supplement because our diets lack the basic nutrients. Others say adequate research is lacking, the government doesn't regulate the industry on the same level as it does pharmaceuticals and some manufacturers make false and outrageous claims.

I am not a certified expert nor do I possess the credentials to offer professional advice. For obvious reasons, my first advice is to direct readers to health care providers. They are the primary care givers. But I know from my experience – and my own research – what works for me.

I take basic vitamin and mineral supplements and fish oil. I take other supplements which I won't disclose in this book. But the supplements

I want to discuss are the ones which have generally helped me. And I insist readers do their own research, consult their physicians and then decide for themselves.

But the point of this chapter is that some supplements seem to have worked for me. I'm not suggesting pills serve or should serve as a magical elixir, although taking certain supplements tends to assist in weight loss. Nearly all of the weight-loss pills marketed today have mixed results and sometimes contrary research.

I generally rely on acai berries, which are relatively inexpensive. For me, acai supplementation – following the manufacturer's suggested daily use – seems to help suppress my appetite. Whether that statement can be documented or whether taking the supplement only functions as a placebo is unimportant. My diet has two planes: psychological and pragmatic. If taking something or doing something works in the long run – and that perhaps is key – then use it, if it's safe and healthy.

Too often dieters toy with unique ideas and complicated programs and see few results. The ongoing thread that hopefully weaves its way through this program is its simplicity and its personalized aspect. The diet has to be easy and it has to be your own. However, as I mentioned earlier, you nonetheless have to have a program. Wishful thinking won't produce lasting or permanent results. Dieting starts in your head, not in your gut or on your butt.

Another pill I've taken – but not regularly – is green coffee beans. The research on this supplement is mixed, but for me it serves to help quicken the digestion process.

Some people in their zeal to find the magic pill go overboard. They buy dozens of bottles and follow the most recent fads hoping something in their stockpile will spark their metabolism to run in overdrive. Short of sprinkling hot sauce or hot pepper on every meal, I've found few natural or nutritional formulas capable of turning up your body's metabolic thermostat.

Successful weight loss programs require determination, discipline and zeal – nothing magical, no secrets. Although the amount of weight some may want to lose seems insurmountable and discouraging, adopting certain principles helps bring you to a new level. When something works and you experience results, you begin to gain confidence. The next chapter deals with the inevitable plateaus that happen along the way and how to approach and deal with them.

Chapter 9 Getting stuck

First the bad news. You will hit plateaus as you descend. Your body sometimes seems to resist the downward spiral of pounds and lays down a set number – this weight and no further. It's discouraging and can easily shred diet programs into pieces. Discouraging news can send you right back to habits and eating patterns that packed the weight on in the first place.

More bad news. Sometimes the plateau lasts for several weeks or even months. Your weight goals seem to move away from you, fading further into that fat future.

Now the good news, hopefully. You have to recognize these plateaus for what they are. They are temporary stops – some longer than others – along the downward trek to your goal. As in a journey, you have to see where you're going and watch for the pitfalls along the way. You have to recognize that the plateaus aren't indicators that your program has failed or that you're destined to return to your starting weight.

The numbers – scrawled boldly across your plateaus – should ideally serve as motivators and make you more determined. It's a battle, and your enemy is the plateau, taunting and teasing you, trying to convince you that this whole idea of losing the high numbers is impossible.

The key, which you have to keep in mind, is recognition. The plateau is temporary. It will not last. Your stubborn adherence to your system will lead you to victory. It's your newfound attitude we discussed earlier. And it's during this stage – the ferocious battle in the mind – that you have to play the hardest ball. Recognize the hard spots, determine to push through and ignore the temptations – and you know what they are – to give in and give up.

You're going down, and that's good.

I've learned to recognize plateaus and how long they last. I've seen them come and go, some lasting a few days, some one or two weeks, some a month or more. But each one eventually succumbs to my determination. I say it again and again. Losing weight is a head game; you lose it in your brain first. It's you against your body. Or, to put it more bluntly, it's the new you – the sleek and slender one you've created in your mind – and the old, fat one you've let develop over time because of bad habits and laziness.

The question is: Who's going to win? That old, fat self may have been around a lot longer; it already has a system in place. When you're hungry, you stuff it until it stops making noise and complaining – with whatever is cheap, easy and often unhealthy. When your feelings are hurt, when you're lonely, when you're celebrating, when you're spending time with family or friends, your body seems to give the order. Eat! Eat! Eat!

Your body is the ruling party. It is the political party that maintains control of your body's chief executive office and both houses of your psychological congress. It is the entity that lays down the law, that dictates solutions to physiological quandaries, that tells you what you should do, why you should do it, and when, which is now!

You have to determine that it's time to overthrow that fat-head regime. You have to recognize – in this campaign – that it may take time to rewire the psychological circuitry, to rewrite your body's biological regulations and to expel with cool and decisive determination the old thought patterns. You have to tell your body who is in charge. Your cravings will no longer be permitted to give the orders (most of the time). They are no longer in charge. You are. While my "bites" program may allow you to satisfy cravings, you have to get hold of the idea that you're the one giving the orders now, not your cravings.

The old order has to submit. And submission – as it relates to your biological demands – always comes with a fight. Depending on how long you've been serving your cravings and your bad eating habits, the old system will not go quietly; it will not leave without a fight and will most of the time return at inconvenient and vulnerable times. That's why you have to adopt a militaristic attitude.

You are the general, and (I'm saying it again) as the general you have to have a plan; you will fail if you rely on disordered, angry will power. The war cannot be won without a strategy. You can only win if you recognize the enemy – your cravings and your old eating habits – and engage in hand-to-hand combat. (Not hand-to-mouth combat.) It's a war, and you won't let up until you settle in at your sleek and slender goal weight. Don't settle for anything less. Don't abandon the vision. Don't step off your plan. Don't retreat. Your mindset: I won't give up. I won't give in. I'll win this battle, no matter how much kicking and screaming the fat monsters do.

Remember. The fat monsters will give in and get quiet if you give them what they want: cheese cake or pizza, for example. But then you've surrendered territory. You've given up ground. Your vision has faded slightly.

You have to recognize the enemy and tell it "no." Then you have to prepare for a fight. The question is: Who will win? Each victory gets easier, each temptation resisted gives more confidence, each old habit squashed establishes new vigor, each splurge rejected lays new psychological wiring in the battlefield of your mind.

That ultimately is what this diet attempts to perform: It attempts to transform you from a fathead to someone who is slim, slender, vibrant and healthy. And that happens mostly between your ears. At first.

In the next and final chapter, I'll be delving deeper, to a more significant and profound level – to your spirit. I warn you now. Some of you may want to get off this bus at this stop of the tour because I will get decidedly spiritual, which is perhaps the most vital element in your trek. If you're staying, here we go. All aboard.

Chapter 10 The gut

I'm going to rely on the Bible to develop a dietary mindset and I'm going to paraphrase certain scriptural passages. This is not a Biblical text, but it does employ Christian principles of the mind, which should follow spiritual directives. The spirit is our origin. It is the center of our being; it directs and shapes our identity.

Our human spirit – in whatever state it's in – is the central force of our existence. We live, move and operate (Acts 17: 28) within the precepts of human spirit and our perceptions of absolute reality. The concepts embedded in the Bible communicate truths to our lives – whether or not we choose to recognize or follow them.

Merely rejecting or choosing to hold different spiritual perspectives doesn't alter the fundamental idea – and the personal reality – of absolute truth.

David in Psalms 139 talks about himself – and about you and me by extension. God's thoughts about you, he says, are precious. The Psalms writer says that God saw him before he was born and that every day of his life was recorded. He said God oversaw the way we were formed – in this case in our mother's womb. David thanks God for making him so wonderful, so complex, so awesome. The Old Testament prophet Jeremiah talks about God knowing him before he was formed in his mother's womb (Jeremiah 1:5).

The tenets displayed in the Bible indicate that we are magnificent creations of God. We were planned for a purpose. We have an eternal destiny to discover and a significance to fill in our individual lives.

So, what went wrong? How did we venture so far off course? How did our lives unravel and how did our bodies fall into such states of disrepair, decay and disease? Why are we sick, fat and tired? And, most of all, how did we become sinners?

The prophets and Biblical writers talk about vision: Without a vision – or a visible, written plan of action – the people perish or lose control. You cannot succeed in life – or with weight loss – without a clear-cut plan. Something has to be established in your life that gives you direction and serves as a guiding force. It has to be something substantial, significant and compelling. And it also has to be a place of passion and desire. Your vision has to provoke zeal and excitement; it has to contain life and wisdom. It must have spiritual animation, an otherworldly aspect that I believe can only be found in the absolute tenets of the Bible.

And to obtain victory in life – and in losing weight – the principles must be absorbed into the fabric of your life. As it is in learning to speak and write a foreign language, you have to learn to inhale the inexhaustible breath of life woven throughout the Bible. Then you have to exhale in the linguistic sense the thought patterns you're acquiring. The way to do that is to find the Biblical principles and make them your own. Adopt them as God's truths spoken into your life and use them as sign posts to guide your life.

Jesus said in Matthew 4:4 that we live by every word that comes from God, and not by food. Later in the same book (12: 34 - 37) Jesus in talking with some religious people says that what comes out of your mouth is an indication of what's already been in you; your words, Jesus says, determine your destiny, in every aspect of your life. Your words – grounded in the truths God established in the Bible and the belief in your spirit – determine your future, your health, your weight, your wellness and how you'll spend eternity.

Jesus said explicitly and without reservation that he is the way, the truth and the life, and that no one can come to the Father, who is God, unless the person accepts Jesus as Savior and Lord. No other options or alternatives exist. That's the starting point – a live relationship with the eternal Creator through a life surrendered to the Bible's Messiah, Jesus.

Solomon in the book of Proverbs says death and life – the quality and extension of our time –

reside in the power of our tongues. In other words, what we say creates the consequences of our lives. We become what we say – in all those idle, negative, complaining words. We are shaped by the words we send into the atmosphere. We are transformed slowly over so many years into a semblance of the linguistic collection of words – that vast pool of sounds – we've uttered.

We ought to take hold of what we say. We have to say what our Creator says about us. We should say about ourselves what David and Jeremiah said about themselves. You have to remind yourself that you are a wonderful creation, a splendid and unique representation of God's handiwork, that you are Divinity's work of art.

You have to stop giving verbal license to your enemy – your cravings, your present appearance, your aches and pains – and start giving your majestic future access to your present tense. And ironically that's done by monitoring what goes in your mouth and what goes out of your mouth. There you have it. That's my secret. In a very large nutshell. Take and eat.

Prologue

Read "Why? Finding the Truth in a Confused World." By William D. Koch

www.ingramcontent.com/pod-product-compliance
Lightning Source LLC
Chambersburg PA
CBHW070345290526
45791CB00003B/1475